ADRENAL RESET DIET FOR BEGINNERS

Delicious Recipes to Cycle Carbs and Proteins for Adrenal Fatigue and Balance Hormones Relieve Stress Also Lose Weight Naturally

By

Dr. Clara Ramsey

Contents

5 | Adrenal Reset Diet for Beginners

Introduction

My Letter to You

Dear Reader,

I would have loved to address you by your first name to Adrenal Reset Diet for Beginners.

But I am doing so if you're holding this book because chances are you've been feeling tired, stressed, and maybe even overwhelmed by the demands of daily life. You may have noticed that no matter how much you diet or exercise, you're not seeing the results you want. You're not alone.

Many people, especially in today's fast-paced world, experience similar struggles—unexplained fatigue, weight gain, difficulty focusing, and mood swings. The truth is, these issues often have less to do with willpower or even calories and more to do with one critical aspect of your health: your adrenal glands.

You might agree with me that adrenal glands play a major role in how your body manages stress, energy levels, and even how you process food. When your adrenals are overworked—whether from chronic stress, poor diet, or lack of sleep—your body becomes unbalanced, and this imbalance can prevent you from living your best life. This is where the Adrenal Reset Diet comes in.

In this book, we're going to take a step-by-step approach to understanding your adrenal health and how simple changes to your diet can help restore balance to your body.

The goal is not just to lose weight but to regain your energy, improve your mood, and feel more in control of your life again.

You'll learn how cycling carbohydrates and proteins throughout the day can positively affect your adrenal glands and reset your body's stress response. This isn't about eliminating entire food groups or making extreme changes; it's about finding the right balance for you.

Whether you're completely new to nutrition or already familiar with the concept of carb cycling, this book will guide you through the process of understanding your adrenals and making sustainable changes that fit your lifestyle.

The information here is grounded in science, and the steps are designed to be easy to follow. You'll have access to practical tools, including meal plans, delicious recipes, and tips for managing stress beyond diet.

Why is this important?

Because when your adrenals are functioning properly, everything else falls into place. You'll sleep better, feel more energized, and start seeing the progress that's been eluding you. You'll not only look better but, more importantly, you'll feel better from the inside out.

Mind you, this book is not about quick fixes. It's about long-term, sustainable health—you have the power to reset your adrenals and take control of your well-being.

By following the Adrenal Reset Diet, you'll equip your body to handle stress, balance your hormones, and thrive in the face of life's demands.

I'm excited for you to begin this journey. Remember, it's not about perfection—it's about progress. Every small step you take toward resetting your adrenals will bring you closer to the health and vitality you deserve.

Here's to your renewed energy and well-being.

Warm regards,

Dr. Clara Ramsey

Chapter One

Why Your Adrenals Matter

The Key to Energy, Weight Loss, and Hormonal Balance

Have you ever felt exhausted, despite getting plenty of rest, or found that your body stubbornly resists weight loss no matter how hard you try?

These frustrating issues might be rooted in a small but powerful pair of glands sitting on top of your kidneys—your adrenal glands. They are your body's energy regulators and stress managers, quietly working behind the scenes to keep everything in balance.

But when they become overworked or under-supported, the impact can ripple through your entire system.

Your adrenals are responsible for producing vital hormones like cortisol, which helps manage your body's response to stress.

When stress levels rise—whether from work, family responsibilities, poor diet, or even lack of sleep, your adrenal glands are forced to work overtime.

This constant demand can throw your hormones out of balance, leading to a cascade of issues like fatigue, stubborn weight gain (especially around the belly), brain fog, and mood swings.

You might wonder, *"What do my adrenals have to do with weight loss?"*

The answer lies in how your body reacts to chronic stress. When your adrenals are on high alert for too long, cortisol levels remain elevated.

This triggers your body to store fat, particularly around your abdomen, as a survival mechanism. Elevated cortisol also disrupts other hormones that regulate hunger and energy, making it harder to feel full or energized.

But here's the good news: when your adrenals are functioning well, you unlock the key to a balanced body. Not only will you find it easier to lose weight, but you'll also enjoy steady energy, improved mood, and overall better health.

It is understanding how to support your adrenals can make all the difference, and that's where the Adrenal Reset Diet comes into play.

The Adrenal Reset Diet

An Overview of the System

So how do we help these overworked adrenal glands get back to doing their job efficiently?

That's the major purpose of the Adrenal Reset Diet. The idea behind this program is simple: by adjusting the types of foods you eat and when you eat them, you can naturally reset your adrenal function, balance your hormones, and restore your body's ability to handle stress.

The core of the Adrenal Reset Diet revolves around a concept called nutrient cycling specifically, cycling carbohydrates and proteins throughout your day to support your body's natural rhythm.

In the morning, your body needs more protein to fuel energy and stabilize blood sugar levels, while carbohydrates in the evening help reduce cortisol and encourage relaxation. This rhythmic approach to eating aligns with your body's natural cycles, allowing your adrenals to rest and recover.

The Adrenal Reset Diet is not restrictive or complicated. It doesn't require cutting out entire food groups or surviving on bland meals. Instead, it's about eating nutrient-rich, whole foods in a way that supports your body's natural balance. By focusing on foods that nourish your adrenals—like lean proteins, healthy fats, and fiber-rich carbohydrates—you can heal from within, without feeling deprived.

It's a sustainable approach that fits into your daily life, giving you the energy you need to thrive, not just survive.

Phases of Adrenal Reset Diet

This diet works in three distinct phases:

Phase 1:

Energy Phase – This phase focuses on supporting your body's energy production by increasing protein intake and minimizing carbs in the early part of the day.

Phase 2:

Balance Phase – In this phase, you'll begin to reintroduce more carbohydrates in the afternoon to balance your blood sugar and cortisol levels.

Phase 3:

Restore Phase – By evening, you'll enjoy more healthy carbs to help your body relax and reset overnight, allowing your adrenals to recover.

It's not just about the food you eat but also about when you eat it. By syncing your meals with your body's natural energy demands, you'll not only feel more vibrant, but you'll also see improvements in weight, sleep, and stress levels.

Understanding Adrenal Fatigue and How It Affects Your Health

If you've been feeling constantly drained or struggling with unexplained symptoms like brain fog or persistent weight gain, you might be dealing with adrenal fatigue. Though it's not widely recognized in conventional medicine, adrenal fatigue is a common problem, especially in today's high-stress world.

Adrenal fatigue happens when your adrenal glands become exhausted from producing too much cortisol over a long period as said earlier. When your body is in a constant state of "fight or flight" mode due to stress, your adrenals never get the chance to rest. Over time, this can lead to cortisol dysregulation, meaning your body either produces too much or too little of this critical hormone.

The signs of adrenal fatigue

Chronic Fatigue: Even after a full night's sleep, you wake up tired and sluggish.

Weight Gain: Particularly around the midsection, which seems impossible to shed.

Sleep Disruptions: Difficulty falling asleep or waking up frequently during the night.

Mood Swings and Irritability: Feeling overwhelmed or anxious for no apparent reason.

Brain Fog: Difficulty concentrating, making decisions, or staying focused.

Left unchecked, adrenal fatigue can wreak havoc on your health, affecting everything from your metabolism to your immune system.

But understanding and addressing adrenal fatigue can lead to profound changes, through proper nutrition, stress management, and lifestyle adjustments, you can restore your adrenal function and take control of your health.

The Adrenal Reset Diet is specifically designed to tackle the root causes of adrenal fatigue. By eating in a way that supports your body's natural rhythms and reduces the stress on your adrenals, you'll begin to feel more energized, focused, and in control of your weight and mood.

The journey to reset your adrenals and restore balance to your life starts with understanding how these tiny glands impact your entire body. With the right approach, including smart food choices and lifestyle changes, you can regain the energy, hormonal balance, and vitality that you deserve.

The Adrenal Reset Diet isn't just another diet—it's a path to long-lasting health and well-being.

Understanding Your Adrenals

Have you ever wondered why some days you feel full of energy, while other days you struggle just to get out of bed?

The answer might lie in a pair of small but incredibly powerful glands that sit quietly atop your kidneys—the adrenal glands. These tiny organs are responsible for helping your body manage stress, regulate energy, and maintain balance in your hormones. Yet, despite their vital role, many of us don't give our adrenal glands much thought—until something goes wrong.

Imagine your adrenal glands as the body's "emergency responders." They jump into action whenever you're faced with a challenge—whether it's a tight deadline, a tough workout, or even an emotional argument.

But, just like any first responder, if they're constantly called into action without a break, they eventually wear out. That's when the trouble begins. Understanding how your adrenals work, and how to support them, can make a world of difference in how you feel every day.

What Are the Adrenal Glands?

Let's start with the basics: *what exactly are the adrenal glands, and why are they so important?*

Your adrenal glands are part of your body's endocrine system, which is responsible for producing and regulating hormones as said earlier. These hormones control everything from your energy levels to your stress response, to how well you sleep at night. Each adrenal gland is made up of two parts: the adrenal cortex (the outer layer) and the adrenal medulla (the inner layer). Together, they work like a team to keep your body balanced.

The Adrenal Cortex: This outer layer produces essential hormones like cortisol and aldosterone. Cortisol is often called the "stress hormone" because it helps your body respond to stress by increasing blood sugar levels, reducing inflammation, and controlling your sleep-wake cycle. Aldosterone, on the other hand, helps regulate your blood pressure and the balance of sodium and potassium in your body.

The Adrenal Medulla: The inner layer of the adrenal gland is where hormones like adrenaline (also known as epinephrine) and noradrenaline (norepinephrine) are produced.

These hormones are responsible for the "fight or flight" response. When you're faced with danger—whether it's a real threat or just a stressful situation—your body releases these hormones to prepare you for action. Your heart rate increases, your muscles get more blood, and your body becomes alert and ready to respond.

In a perfect world, your adrenal glands would only be called upon in truly stressful situations, allowing them to function optimally and give your body the energy it needs when it really matters. But in reality, the modern world often keeps us in a state of chronic stress.

Whether it's work deadlines, financial worries, or constant screen time, our adrenal glands are constantly producing cortisol and adrenaline, keeping our bodies on high alert. Over time, this can lead to adrenal fatigue, where the adrenal glands struggle to keep up with the demands placed on them.

Here's the tricky part: your adrenal glands don't just respond to emotional stress. Physical stress—like poor diet, lack of sleep, and even over-exercising—can also tax your adrenals.

When the adrenals are overworked, it can lead to hormonal imbalances that affect everything from your weight to your mood.

The Impact of Adrenal Health on Your Everyday Life

When your adrenal glands are functioning well, they provide the right amount of hormones to keep you energized and balanced throughout the day.

However, if your adrenal glands are constantly overworked, you may experience symptoms that can be easily mistaken for something else, like chronic fatigue or burnout.

Common signs that your adrenal glands might be struggling include:

Unexplained Fatigue: Even after a good night's sleep, you wake up feeling tired and sluggish, often reaching for caffeine or sugar to get through the day.

Weight Gain, Especially Around the Belly: This is due to the constant high levels of cortisol, which prompts your body to store fat, particularly in the abdomen.

Sleep Disruptions: You may find it hard to fall asleep or wake up in the middle of the night, wired but tired.

Mood Swings and Anxiety: Constant stress can lead to emotional highs and lows, making it hard to manage your mood.

Low Energy and Lack of Focus: Brain fog and difficulty concentrating are common, especially in the afternoons.

It's easy to blame these symptoms on aging or the demands of modern life, but often, it's your adrenal glands waving a white flag, signaling they need help. Fortunately, by making some strategic changes—like adjusting your diet, managing stress, and getting enough rest—you can support your adrenal glands and help them recover.

How to Support Your Adrenal Glands

The good news is that your adrenal glands are resilient, and with the right support, they can bounce back. By nourishing your body with the right foods, managing stress more effectively, and following the principles of the Adrenal Reset Diet, you can help restore balance and function to these crucial glands.

Here are a few key steps to support your adrenal health:

Eat a Balanced Diet: Focus on nutrient-dense foods that provide sustained energy throughout the day. Lean proteins, healthy fats, and slow-digesting carbohydrates can help keep blood sugar stable, preventing the spikes and crashes that strain your adrenal glands.

Cycle Your Nutrients: As you'll learn in the Adrenal Reset Diet, cycling carbohydrates and proteins throughout the day can support your adrenal glands' natural rhythm, giving them the rest they need to function optimally.

Prioritize Rest and Recovery: Your adrenal glands need time to recover. Getting quality sleep, taking breaks during the day, and managing your workload are all essential steps to reducing stress on your adrenals.

Practice Stress-Management Techniques: Incorporate relaxation techniques like deep breathing, meditation, or yoga into your routine. These practices help lower cortisol levels, giving your adrenal glands a much-needed break.

By understanding the important role your adrenal glands play in regulating energy, stress, and hormones, you can start taking steps to support them. With the right approach, you'll not only improve your adrenal health but also enjoy more energy, better sleep, and a more balanced life.

The journey to adrenal health begins with awareness, and now that you understand how vital these little glands are, you're one step closer to resetting your body for good.

The Role of Adrenals in Your Body's Stress Response

Your adrenal glands are like the body's command center for handling stress.

Picture them as your built-in crisis managers, always ready to respond to challenges—whether it's a sudden scare, a looming deadline, or even intense exercise. The adrenals, a small, triangle-shaped glands that might seem unassuming, they play a critical role in how your body reacts to everyday stressors.

At the heart of this response is a hormone called cortisol, which is often referred to as the "stress hormone." However, the adrenals don't just stop at cortisol. They also produce adrenaline (or epinephrine), which is responsible for the immediate fight-or-flight reaction you experience when faced with danger. Together, these hormones allow your body to either confront a threat head-on or retreat to safety.

So, how does it all work?

When your brain perceives a stressor—whether it's physical, emotional, or mental—it signals your adrenal glands to release hormones like cortisol and adrenaline.

These hormones prepare your body for action by:

Increasing Heart Rate: Adrenaline spikes your heart rate, pumping more blood to your muscles so you're ready for quick movement.

Elevating Blood Sugar: Cortisol boosts blood sugar levels, providing your body with the quick energy it needs to respond to the stressor.

Suppressing Non-Essential Functions: During a crisis, your body temporarily shuts down processes like digestion and immune responses to conserve energy for immediate survival.

This system is brilliant for short-term stress, such as reacting quickly to avoid a car accident or gearing up for an important presentation.

However, when stress becomes chronic—like constant work pressure, financial worries, or emotional turmoil—your adrenal glands remain in overdrive, constantly pumping out cortisol. This prolonged stress response can wear down your body, leading to what is known as adrenal fatigue.

Chapter Two

Signs and Symptoms of Adrenal Fatigue

Adrenal fatigue is a condition where your adrenal glands become overworked and unable to keep up with the continuous demand for cortisol.

Think of it like a muscle that gets overused: at first, it performs well, but after too much strain, it weakens and can no longer function properly.

When your adrenals are tired, your body struggles to manage stress, and you start to experience a range of symptoms that can affect nearly every aspect of your life.

Here are the most common signs and symptoms of adrenal fatigue:

Chronic Fatigue

Feeling exhausted all the time, no matter how much rest you get, is one of the hallmark signs of adrenal fatigue.

You might wake up in the morning feeling unrefreshed, and as the day progresses, even simple tasks feel overwhelming. Some people describe it as "hitting a wall" in the afternoon when energy levels plummet.

Sleep Issues

Adrenal fatigue often disrupts your sleep cycle, making it difficult to fall asleep at night or causing you to wake up frequently.

Even if you do manage to get enough hours of sleep, the quality of that sleep is often poor, leaving you groggy the next day.

Unexplained Weight Gain

One of the most frustrating symptoms of adrenal fatigue is unexplained weight gain, especially around the abdomen.

High levels of cortisol prompt your body to store fat, particularly visceral fat, which is stored around your organs and is harder to lose.

Cravings for Salt and Sugar

Because adrenal fatigue disrupts your body's ability to regulate blood sugar, you may find yourself craving sugary snacks or salty foods throughout the day.

These cravings are your body's way of trying to boost energy levels quickly, but they often lead to a cycle of highs and lows in energy.

Brain Fog and Difficulty Concentrating

Do you find it hard to focus or remember details? Brain fog is a common symptom of adrenal fatigue. The constant production of cortisol can interfere with brain function,

33 | Adrenal Reset Diet for Beginners

making it difficult to concentrate, think clearly, or retain information.

Mood Swings, Anxiety, and Irritability

When your body is under stress for long periods, it's not just physical exhaustion that sets in—emotional exhaustion follows.

You may feel more anxious, irritable, or prone to mood swings than usual. Small things that wouldn't normally bother you suddenly feel overwhelming.

Weakened Immune System

Cortisol, in healthy amounts, has an anti-inflammatory effect on the body. But when cortisol levels are consistently high due to chronic stress, your immune system becomes suppressed, making you more susceptible to infections and illnesses like colds or the flu.

Low Libido

Hormonal imbalances caused by adrenal fatigue often affect your reproductive health. Women may experience irregular menstrual cycles or decreased interest in intimacy, while men may face challenges with maintaining a healthy libido.

This is because cortisol interferes with the production of sex hormones like estrogen and testosterone.

Dizziness and Lightheadedness

Adrenal fatigue can also impact blood pressure. You may feel lightheaded or dizzy, particularly when standing up too quickly, as your body struggles to maintain proper blood flow and pressure regulation.

Increased Reliance on Stimulants

Many people with adrenal fatigue find themselves reaching for more caffeine or sugar throughout the day just to feel functional.

35 | Adrenal Reset Diet for Beginners

While these stimulants may provide a short-term boost, they only further deplete your adrenals in the long run, creating a vicious cycle of fatigue and dependence.

The Vicious Cycle of Adrenal Fatigue

What makes adrenal fatigue particularly challenging is its cyclical nature. When your adrenal glands are overworked, you become more susceptible to stress, which further taxes the adrenals. As the fatigue deepens, you may find yourself relying on sugar, caffeine, or other quick fixes to boost your energy, but these only contribute to long-term hormonal imbalances. Eventually, this vicious cycle can lead to burnout, where you feel like your body is simply running on empty.

Fortunately, there's a way out of this cycle. The first step is recognizing the symptoms and understanding that adrenal fatigue is your body's way of signaling that it needs support.

By focusing on proper nutrition, stress management, and lifestyle changes—like following the Adrenal Reset Diet—you can give your adrenal glands the break they desperately need, allowing them to recover and function properly again.

By understanding the role your adrenal glands play in your stress response and recognizing the signs of adrenal fatigue, you can take the necessary steps to regain control over your energy, mood, and overall health. It's about working with your body's natural systems, rather than against them, to restore balance and vitality.

How Stress and Diet Impact Adrenal Health

We've all experienced stress, it's unavoidable. *But did you know that how you manage it, and what you eat, can significantly impact your adrenal glands and overall well-being?*

37 | Adrenal Reset Diet for Beginners

Am sure you don't know, but I can tell you that your adrenal health is at the intersection of stress and nutrition. Stress isn't just something you feel mentally or emotionally; it has real, physical effects on your body, especially on your adrenal glands.

At the same time, the foods you choose can either support your adrenals or make them work harder.

Let's break it down. Understanding how stress and diet influence adrenal function is key to maintaining balanced energy, better mood, and better resilience to the demands of life.

The Stress-Hormone Connection

Think about how your body reacts to stress. Maybe your heart races, your muscles tense, or your thoughts speed up. Behind the scenes, your adrenal glands are hard at work, orchestrating these responses by releasing a powerful mix of hormones—primarily cortisol and adrenaline. This hormonal surge is what prepares your body for the classic "fight-or-flight" reaction.

Here's a simple example: You're stuck in traffic, late for an important meeting. Your brain registers this as a stressful situation and sends a message to your adrenal glands. In response, your adrenals release cortisol and adrenaline, pumping up your heart rate and raising your blood sugar so you have the energy and focus to deal with the stress. This is your body's way of getting you through tough moments.

Cortisol, often called the "stress hormone," is key here. In small amounts, it helps your body respond to stress effectively. It's involved in everything from regulating your metabolism to controlling your sleep-wake cycle. But when you're under constant stress, cortisol levels remain elevated for longer periods.

Over time, this chronic stress wears down your adrenals, leading to what's known as adrenal fatigue.

The problem? Your adrenal glands weren't designed to be in overdrive all the time. When you're always stressed—whether from work pressures, financial strain, or even emotional stress—your body keeps pumping out cortisol. This can lead to a cascade of health issues: weight gain (especially around the belly), mood swings, fatigue, and even sleep problems.

Essentially, your body is stuck in survival mode, and your adrenal glands become exhausted.

Chronic Stress: A Silent Saboteur

Chronic stress doesn't just affect your energy levels; it impacts your whole system:

Immune Function: Prolonged cortisol production weakens the immune system, leaving you more susceptible to illnesses.

Digestive Health: High cortisol levels can interfere with digestion, leading to bloating, indigestion, or even more severe gastrointestinal issues.

Hormonal Imbalance: Your adrenals don't work alone. They're part of a larger hormonal network, and when cortisol is consistently high, it can throw off the balance of other key hormones like insulin, estrogen, and testosterone.

In essence, stress is a trigger that can throw your entire system out of balance if it's not managed effectively, and here's where diet steps in as an essential factor in maintaining healthy adrenal function.

The Influence of Nutrition on Adrenal Function

Just as stress can overwork your adrenal glands, what you eat can either support or strain them. In fact, diet plays a vital role in helping your adrenal glands manage stress more effectively and recover from the effects of adrenal fatigue.

Blood Sugar Balance: The Adrenals' Best Friend

One of cortisol's main jobs is to regulate your blood sugar levels. When blood sugar drops too low, the adrenal glands release cortisol to raise it back to normal.

If your diet is loaded with refined carbs and sugars—like pastries, candy, or soda—your blood sugar spikes and crashes frequently. This yo-yo effect forces your adrenal glands to work overtime to keep your blood sugar stable.

Over time, this constant demand for cortisol to stabilize blood sugar wears down your adrenals, contributing to fatigue.

The solution? Stabilizing your blood sugar through balanced meals and snacks that include protein, healthy fats, and fiber can give your adrenals the break they need.

Here's how a balanced meal can help:

- Proteins (like lean meats, beans, or eggs) provide steady energy and help repair cells.
- Healthy Fats (from sources like avocado, nuts, and olive oil) give your body long-lasting fuel without the spikes in blood sugar.
- Fiber (found in vegetables, whole grains, and legumes) slows down digestion, ensuring your blood sugar stays steady for longer periods.

Nutrient Deficiencies and Adrenal Fatigue

Your adrenal glands also depend on certain vitamins and minerals to function optimally. Without these key nutrients, your adrenals struggle to produce the right amount of hormones and manage stress effectively.

Here are some key nutrients that support adrenal health:

- **Vitamin C:** Your adrenals contain the highest concentration of vitamin C in your entire body. It's essential for producing cortisol and other adrenal hormones.
- Foods like bell peppers, citrus fruits, and broccoli are great sources.
- **Magnesium:** This mineral helps regulate the stress response and supports the relaxation of muscles and nerves.
- Dark leafy greens, nuts, and seeds are excellent sources of magnesium.
- **B Vitamins:** Especially B5 (pantothenic acid) and B6, which are directly involved in adrenal hormone production.

- Whole grains, beans, nuts, and animal proteins are rich in these essential vitamins.
- *Zinc:* This mineral supports immune function and helps balance cortisol levels.
- Foods like shellfish, beef, and pumpkin seeds provide a good dose of zinc.

When you're chronically stressed, your body uses up these nutrients faster than usual. Over time, nutrient depletion makes it harder for your adrenals to keep up with the demands placed on them, leading to feelings of burnout, fatigue, and even immune dysfunction.

Caffeine and Sugar

The Hidden Stressors on the Adrenals

Let's talk about two common dietary habits that can secretly sabotage your adrenal health: caffeine and sugar.

45 | Adrenal Reset Diet for Beginners

While that morning cup of coffee might feel like an energy booster, caffeine actually stimulates the release of adrenaline, this adds more strain on your adrenal glands. If you're already feeling fatigued, relying on caffeine for energy can create a vicious cycle where your adrenal glands never get the rest they need.

Similarly, sugar creates sharp spikes and crashes in blood sugar, leading to more cortisol production. The more sugar you eat, the harder your adrenal glands have to work to stabilize your blood sugar.

Supporting Your Adrenal Health Through Diet

So, what's the best way to support your adrenal glands?

It starts with eating a nutrient-rich, balanced diet that keeps your blood sugar stable and provides the essential vitamins and minerals your adrenals need to function properly.

Here are a few tips:

Eat Regular, Balanced Meals: Don't skip meals. Your adrenals need steady fuel throughout the day. Include proteins, healthy fats, and slow-digesting carbohydrates (like whole grains or vegetables) in each meal.

Snack Smart: When you feel your energy dipping, reach for nutrient-dense snacks like a handful of nuts, a boiled egg, or veggies with hummus. Avoid sugary treats that will only lead to a crash later.

Hydrate Well: Dehydration puts extra stress on your adrenals. Drink water consistently throughout the day and consider adding a pinch of sea salt to your water for an added boost of electrolytes, which can help balance your energy.

Reduce Stimulants: If you rely heavily on caffeine or sugary snacks, try cutting back gradually to give your adrenals a break. Opt for herbal teas or decaf options instead.

Focus on Whole, Unprocessed Foods: The closer your food is to its natural state, the better it will be for your adrenal health. Processed foods tend to contain added sugars, unhealthy fats, and artificial ingredients that can further stress your body.

Let me tell you, stress and diet are two sides of the same coin when it comes to adrenal health. While stress can overwork your adrenals, the right diet can give them the support they need to recover and function at their best.

By eating nutrient-rich foods, stabilizing your blood sugar, and cutting down on stimulants like caffeine and sugar, you'll be well on your way to improving both your adrenal health and overall well-being.

Chapter Three

The Science Behind the Adrenal Reset Diet

If you've ever felt stuck in a cycle of exhaustion, cravings, and stress, you're not alone. The Adrenal Reset Diet was created to address exactly that—by giving your adrenal glands the support they need to function optimally and helping you regain control over your energy, metabolism, and mood.

But what's the science behind this diet, and how does it work to reset your adrenal glands?

At its core, the Adrenal Reset Diet revolves around the concept of nutrient cycling, which is designed to balance the hormones that govern your stress response, metabolism, and even your ability to lose weight. The beauty of this approach is that it works with your body's natural rhythms instead of fighting against them.

By strategically cycling carbohydrates and proteins throughout the day, you can shift your body from "survival mode" (where stress hormones dominate) to "thriving mode" (where your body feels calm, energized, and resilient).

Let's break down the key principles and the science behind this revolutionary approach.

The Power of Nutrient Cycling

Nutrient cycling is exactly what it sounds like—alternating the types of nutrients you consume throughout the day to optimize your hormone levels and support adrenal health.

But this isn't just about eating healthier foods (although that's a big part of it). It's about timing your intake of carbohydrates, proteins, and fats to work in sync with your body's natural rhythms.

50 | Adrenal Reset Diet for Beginners

Think of your body as having two modes: daytime mode and nighttime mode.

Daytime mode is your active, high-energy state. During this time, your body naturally produces more cortisol, the hormone that helps you stay alert and focused. In the morning and early afternoon, you want to support cortisol production with proteins and healthy fats, which provide sustained energy without spiking blood sugar.

Nighttime mode is when your body shifts into repair and recovery. As the day winds down, your cortisol levels should naturally decrease and the hormone melatonin takes over to help you relax and prepare for sleep.

This is the perfect time to consume carbohydrates, which encourage the production of serotonin (the feel-good hormone), helping to lower cortisol and ease you into restful sleep.

51 | Adrenal Reset Diet for Beginners

By cycling the types of nutrients you eat at different times of the day, you essentially reset your body's stress response, allowing your adrenals to recover and function more efficiently.

Carb and Protein Cycling:

One of the central components of the Adrenal Reset Diet is carbohydrate and protein cycling. It's a method that helps you manipulate the levels of key hormones—especially cortisol and insulin—in a way that supports adrenal health, weight management, and overall well-being.

Here's how it works:

Morning (High Protein, Low Carb)

In the morning, your cortisol levels are naturally at their highest. This is your body's way of helping you wake up, stay alert, and handle the demands of the day.

To support this, the diet recommends starting the day with a meal that's high in protein and healthy fats, while keeping carbs to a minimum.

Why? Protein helps to stabilize blood sugar and provides a slow, steady release of energy throughout the day. This prevents the energy crashes and sugar cravings that often result from a high-carb breakfast.

Think eggs with avocado, a protein smoothie with nut butter, or a veggie omelet with olive oil.

Afternoon (Balanced Protein and Carbs)

By midday, your cortisol levels should start to dip slightly as your body shifts gears from peak alertness to a more moderate energy level. This is the time to balance protein and carbohydrates in your meal.

Adding a moderate amount of healthy carbs at lunch helps to prevent an afternoon energy slump by keeping blood sugar steady without overstimulating cortisol production. You still want a good amount of protein to stay satisfied and focused.

Think: grilled chicken with quinoa and veggies, or a salad with salmon and sweet potato.

Evening (Higher Carb, Lower Protein)

In the evening, your goal is to lower cortisol levels and prepare your body for rest and recovery. This is when you'll want to include more carbohydrates in your meal, which can help calm the nervous system by boosting serotonin and reducing stress hormones.

Don't worry about carbs causing weight gain here. When consumed at the right time, healthy carbohydrates can actually help with fat loss by promoting a balanced cortisol curve and better sleep.

Think: brown rice with stir-fried veggies, or a sweet potato with a drizzle of olive oil and roasted vegetables.

This daily rhythm of nutrient cycling encourages your body to produce the right hormones at the right time, which leads to better energy, improved mood, and sustainable weight management.

By synchronizing your eating habits with your body's natural cycles, you're essentially helping your adrenal glands recover from the constant demands of modern life.

Why Cycling is Essential for Adrenal Health

The real magic of the Adrenal Reset Diet lies in the power of cycling—because your adrenal glands thrive on balance. Chronic stress, poor diet, and sleep deprivation throw this balance out of whack, leading to adrenal fatigue, hormone imbalances, and a cascade of other health issues.

55 | Adrenal Reset Diet for Beginners

So, why is cycling your nutrients essential for adrenal health? Here's why:

Preventing Adrenal Overload

When your diet is high in refined carbohydrates or sugar, your blood sugar spikes and crashes throughout the day, causing your adrenal glands to release more and more cortisol to keep up. This constant demand on your adrenals can lead to burnout over time.

By strategically timing your carb intake—loading up on proteins in the morning and reserving healthy carbs for later in the day—you prevent these sharp fluctuations in blood sugar, giving your adrenal glands a break.

Supporting Natural Cortisol Rhythms

Cortisol isn't inherently bad—in fact, you need it to function. But it's the timing of cortisol that matters. You want cortisol levels to be high in the morning when you need energy and focus, and low in the evening when it's time to unwind. Carb and protein cycling supports this natural rhythm, helping to reset your body's cortisol curve.

When cortisol is balanced, you'll experience better sleep, more stable energy, and reduced cravings for unhealthy foods.

Optimizing Hormonal Balance

Your adrenal glands don't work alone. They're part of a complex hormonal system that includes insulin (which controls blood sugar), melatonin (which regulates sleep), and even sex hormones like estrogen and testosterone.

When cortisol levels are too high for too long, it throws this entire system out of balance.

Nutrient cycling helps keep these hormones in check by providing the right nutrients at the right time. For instance, eating carbs in the evening boosts serotonin, which leads to more melatonin production—helping you sleep better and wake up feeling refreshed.

Promoting Fat Loss and Muscle Maintenance

One of the most frustrating effects of adrenal fatigue is weight gain, especially around the midsection. When your body is in constant "fight-or-flight" mode, it stores fat as a survival mechanism.

Carb and protein cycling can help reverse this process by stabilizing insulin levels and encouraging your body to burn fat for fuel, rather than storing it.

Plus, the high-protein, low-carb approach in the morning helps preserve muscle mass, which is crucial for maintaining a healthy metabolism.

the Adrenal Reset Diet is more than just a weight-loss program—it's a comprehensive approach to healing your adrenals, balancing your hormones, and restoring your energy.

By using the science of nutrient cycling, you can support your body's natural rhythms, prevent burnout, and unlock the energy you need to thrive.

Chapter Four

Your Body's Energy Rhythm

Have you ever noticed how your energy levels ebb and flow throughout the day?

One moment you're bouncing with enthusiasm, and the next, you're struggling to keep your eyes open. This isn't just a coincidence; it's your body's natural energy rhythm at work.

Understanding this rhythm is key to optimizing your health and well-being.

Your body follows a daily cycle known as the circadian rhythm, a 24-hour internal clock that regulates various physiological processes, including sleep-wake cycles, hormone production, and metabolism. This rhythm is influenced by light, temperature, and your daily activities, and it dictates when you feel most alert or sleepy.

By aligning your diet with this natural rhythm, you can harness your body's peak energy periods and support overall health.

Adapting Your Diet to Your Circadian Rhythm

Imagine your body as a finely tuned orchestra, where each part plays its role in harmony with the rest. The circadian rhythm acts as the conductor, setting the tempo for everything from hormone release to energy expenditure.

Adapting your diet to this rhythm can enhance your vitality, improve sleep quality, and support metabolic health.

Morning: Energize and Stabilize

In the morning, your circadian rhythm sets the stage for a surge in cortisol, the hormone responsible for waking you up and boosting your alertness.

To complement this natural rise, start your day with a breakfast that stabilizes blood sugar and provides sustained energy. Focus on high-protein and healthy fats that keep you full and energized throughout the day.

Protein (like eggs, Greek yogurt, or tofu) provides a steady release of energy and prevents the sugar crashes that can occur with high-carb breakfasts.

Healthy fats (such as avocados, nuts, and seeds) help maintain stable blood sugar levels and support overall hormone function.

By eating a balanced breakfast, you align with your body's natural cortisol peak, setting a positive tone for the rest of your day.

Afternoon: Sustain and Balance

As the day progresses, your cortisol levels gradually decline, and your body shifts to a different phase of energy regulation. In the afternoon, aim for meals that balance protein and carbohydrates. This balance ensures steady energy without overwhelming your body with excess stress or blood sugar fluctuations.

Complex carbs (like quinoa, sweet potatoes, or whole grains) provide long-lasting energy without causing sharp spikes in blood sugar.

Lean protein (such as chicken, beans, or lentils) keeps you satisfied and supports muscle function.

This balanced approach helps maintain steady energy levels and prevents the mid-afternoon slump that many people experience.

Evening: Relax and Recover

In the evening, your body prepares for rest, and cortisol levels should naturally decrease. To support this transition, focus on carbohydrates in your dinner to promote relaxation and better sleep.

Complex carbs (like brown rice, whole-grain pasta, or a small serving of fruit) can boost serotonin levels, which helps reduce cortisol and prepare your body for a restful night.

Avoid heavy, high-fat, or overly spicy meals close to bedtime, as these can interfere with sleep quality and digestion. Instead, opt for a light, nourishing meal that supports relaxation and recovery.

How to Balance Carbs and Proteins Based on Stress Levels

Stress is an inevitable part of life, but how you manage your diet in response to how you can make a significant difference. Your stress levels can affect how your body processes nutrients, and adjusting your carb and protein intake based on these levels is crucial for maintaining energy and hormonal balance.

High Stress Levels: Prioritize Balance

When stress levels are high, your body produces more cortisol and experiences increased blood sugar fluctuations. To counteract this:

Increase protein intake to help stabilize blood sugar and reduce cravings. Protein-rich foods like lean meats, eggs, and legumes can help keep you feeling full and balanced.

Moderate carbohydrate intake and focus on complex carbs that have a low glycemic index (like sweet potatoes, oats, and beans). This helps prevent rapid spikes and crashes in blood sugar.

Low to Moderate Stress Levels: Optimize Energy

During periods of lower stress, your body can handle a more balanced approach to carbs and proteins. You can enjoy a varied diet that includes:

65 | Adrenal Reset Diet for Beginners

A good mix of proteins and carbohydrates in each meal. This helps support steady energy levels and keeps your metabolism running smoothly.

Healthy fats (such as those found in nuts, seeds, and olive oil) to support overall hormonal health.

By maintaining this balance, you can enjoy sustained energy throughout the day and support your body's natural rhythms without overloading your stress response.

While understanding and adapting to your body's energy rhythm is a powerful tool in achieving optimal health.

By aligning your diet with your circadian rhythm, you can enhance your energy levels, support hormonal balance, and improve your overall well-being.

Balancing your intake of carbohydrates and proteins based on stress levels ensures that your body functions at its best, no matter what life throws your way.

So, the next time you plan your meals, remember: timing and balance are key. By syncing your diet with your body's natural rhythms, you're not just eating for health—you're eating in harmony with yourself.

Chapter Five

Foods to Focus On

1. Lean Proteins: Proteins are vital for stabilizing blood sugar and supporting adrenal function. They help manage stress hormones and repair tissues.

Examples: Chicken breast, turkey, fish, tofu, legumes (beans, lentils), and eggs.

Why: Protein helps prevent energy crashes and keeps you feeling full longer, which can reduce the strain on your adrenals.

2. Healthy Fats: Fats are essential for hormone production and help in absorbing fat-soluble vitamins. They also provide long-lasting energy without spiking blood sugar.

Examples: Avocados, nuts (almonds, walnuts), seeds (chia, flax), olive oil, and fatty fish (salmon, mackerel).

Why: Healthy fats support adrenal health by maintaining stable energy levels and hormone balance.

3. Complex Carbohydrates: Carbs are an important source of energy, especially when consumed in their complex form, which releases glucose slowly into the bloodstream.

Examples: Whole grains (brown rice, quinoa, oats), starchy vegetables (sweet potatoes, butternut squash), and legumes.

Why: They provide sustained energy and help manage blood sugar levels, reducing stress on the adrenals.

4. Vegetables: Rich in vitamins, minerals, and antioxidants, vegetables support overall health and reduce inflammation.

Examples: Leafy greens (spinach, kale), cruciferous vegetables (broccoli, Brussels sprouts), and colorful veggies (bell peppers, carrots).

Why: They provide essential nutrients and antioxidants that help reduce stress and support adrenal health.

5. Fruits: Fruits are a great source of vitamins, minerals, and fiber, which are important for energy and overall health.

Examples: Berries (blueberries, strawberries), apples, oranges, and bananas (in moderation).

Why: They offer natural sweetness and a dose of essential vitamins and minerals. Opt for fruits with a low glycemic index to avoid blood sugar spikes.

6. Hydrating Foods and Drinks: Staying hydrated is crucial for adrenal health.

Adequate hydration supports energy levels and helps manage stress.

Examples: Water, herbal teas (chamomile, peppermint), and hydrating fruits and vegetables (cucumbers, watermelon).

Why: Proper hydration aids in maintaining electrolyte balance and supports overall bodily functions.

7. Nutrient-Dense Foods: These foods are packed with vitamins and minerals that support adrenal function and overall health.

Examples: Nuts and seeds, leafy greens, berries, and foods rich in vitamin C (citrus fruits, bell peppers).

Why: Nutrient-dense foods provide essential vitamins and minerals needed for optimal adrenal function and stress management.

Foods to Avoid

1. Refined Sugars: Sugary foods and beverages can cause rapid spikes and crashes in blood sugar, leading to increased cortisol production and adrenal strain.

Examples: Candy, pastries, sugary cereals, soda, and energy drinks.

Why: High sugar intake can lead to energy crashes, weight gain, and increased stress on the adrenals.

2. Processed Foods: These often contain high levels of unhealthy fats, sugars, and artificial additives that can negatively impact adrenal health and overall well-being.

Examples: Fast food, packaged snacks, frozen meals, and processed meats.

Why: Processed foods are typically low in nutrients and high in ingredients that can disrupt hormonal balance and increase stress.

3. Caffeine: While caffeine can provide a temporary boost, excessive consumption can overstimulate the adrenal glands and lead to increased cortisol levels.

Examples: Coffee, caffeinated teas, energy drinks, and some sodas.

Why: High caffeine intake can disrupt sleep patterns, increase anxiety, and lead to adrenal fatigue.

4. Refined Carbohydrates: These can cause rapid blood sugar spikes and contribute to inflammation and weight gain.

Examples: White bread, pastries, sugary snacks, and other products made with refined flour.

Why: Refined carbs can lead to blood sugar imbalances and stress the adrenal glands.

5. High-Sodium Foods: Excessive salt can contribute to high blood pressure and disrupt fluid balance in the body, adding stress to the adrenal glands.

Examples: Processed and canned foods, salty snacks, and fast food.

Why: High sodium intake can lead to fluid imbalances and stress the body's overall system, including the adrenals.

6. Trans Fats and Unhealthy Oils: These can promote inflammation and negatively affect hormone production.

Examples: Margarine, fried foods, and foods made with hydrogenated oils.

Why: Trans fats can lead to increased inflammation and hormone imbalances, which can strain the adrenal glands.

7. Alcohol: Alcohol can disrupt sleep, impact blood sugar levels, and stress the liver and adrenals.

Examples: Beer, wine, spirits, and mixed alcoholic drinks.

Why: Alcohol consumption can interfere with sleep patterns, blood sugar regulation, and overall adrenal health.

Choosing the right foods can significantly impact your adrenal health and overall well-being. Focusing on nutrient-dense, whole foods while avoiding refined sugars, processed foods, and excessive caffeine or alcohol can help your body function at its best. By aligning your diet with your body's natural rhythms and supporting your adrenal glands with balanced nutrition, you set yourself up for sustained energy, better mood, and overall vitality.

30-Day Adrenal Reset Meal Plan

Here's a comprehensive 30-day meal plan designed to support adrenal health. Each day features balanced meals and snacks, emphasizing nutrient-rich foods, strategic carb and protein cycling, and variety to keep the plan engaging. Leftovers are used to minimize food waste and save time.

Week 1

Day 1

Breakfast: Scrambled eggs with spinach and avocado

Lunch: Grilled chicken salad with mixed greens, cherry tomatoes, and olive oil vinaigrette

Dinner: Baked salmon with quinoa and steamed broccoli

Snack: Handful of almonds

Day 2

Breakfast: Greek yogurt with berries and chia seeds

Lunch: Lentil soup with a side of mixed greens

Dinner: Turkey and vegetable stir-fry with brown rice

Snack: Carrot sticks with hummus

Day 3

Breakfast: Smoothie with spinach, banana, protein powder, and almond milk

Lunch: Quinoa and black bean salad with bell peppers and lime dressing

Dinner: Chicken breast with sweet potato and green beans

Snack: Apple slices with almond butter

Day 4

Breakfast: Overnight oats with chia seeds, nuts, and fresh berries

Lunch: Turkey wrap with whole-grain tortilla, lettuce, and avocado

Dinner: Baked cod with roasted Brussels sprouts and wild rice

Snack: Greek yogurt with a drizzle of honey

Day 5

Breakfast: Omelet with mushrooms, onions, and bell peppers

Lunch: Chickpea and vegetable curry with cauliflower rice

Dinner: Grilled shrimp skewers with zucchini noodles and a side salad

Snack: A handful of walnuts

Day 6

Breakfast: Smoothie bowl with spinach, frozen berries, and granola

Lunch: Spinach and feta-stuffed chicken breast with a side of roasted sweet potatoes

Dinner: Beef and vegetable stew with a side of steamed green beans

Snack: Celery sticks with almond butter

Day 7

Breakfast: Chia pudding topped with kiwi and coconut flakes

Lunch: Mixed bean salad with tomatoes, cucumbers, and balsamic dressing

Dinner: Grilled turkey burgers with a side of sautéed spinach and quinoa

Snack: Cottage cheese with pineapple chunks

Week 2

Day 8

Breakfast: Avocado toast on whole-grain bread with a poached egg

Lunch: Chicken and vegetable soup with a side salad

Dinner: Baked tilapia with roasted carrots and brown rice

Snack: Mixed nuts

Day 9

Breakfast: Greek yogurt smoothie with spinach, mango, and protein powder

Lunch: Falafel wrap with hummus and a side of tabbouleh

Dinner: Stuffed bell peppers with ground turkey and cauliflower rice

Snack: Orange slices

Day 10

Breakfast: Egg muffins with spinach and feta

Lunch: Quinoa and chickpea salad with cucumber, tomato, and a lemon dressing

Dinner: Grilled pork chops with a side of mashed sweet potatoes and sautéed kale

Snack: Fresh berries

Day 11

Breakfast: Overnight chia pudding with almond milk and fresh fruit

Lunch: Tuna salad with mixed greens and a side of whole-grain crackers

Dinner: Spaghetti squash with marinara sauce and turkey meatballs

Snack: Sliced bell peppers with guacamole

Day 12

Breakfast: Smoothie with kale, apple, protein powder, and unsweetened almond milk

Lunch: Chicken Caesar salad (without croutons)

Dinner: Baked haddock with a side of roasted Brussels sprouts and wild rice

Snack: Handful of sunflower seeds

Day 13

Breakfast: Banana and almond butter smoothie

Lunch: Vegetable and tofu stir-fry with brown rice

Dinner: Beef fajitas with bell peppers and onions, served with a side of guacamole

Snack: Sliced cucumber with hummus

Day 14

Breakfast: Almond flour pancakes with fresh berries

Lunch: Lentil and vegetable stew with a side of mixed greens

Dinner: Grilled chicken thighs with roasted sweet potatoes and green beans

Snack: Greek yogurt with a sprinkle of nuts

Week 3

Day 15

Breakfast: Smoothie bowl with spinach, avocado, and a handful of granola

Lunch: Turkey and avocado lettuce wraps with a side of sliced tomatoes

Dinner: Baked salmon with a side of quinoa and steamed broccoli

Snack: Handful of almonds

Day 16

Breakfast: Scrambled eggs with tomatoes and spinach

Lunch: Chickpea salad with mixed greens and a lemon-tahini dressing

Dinner: Stuffed zucchini boats with ground beef and cauliflower rice

Snack: Fresh apple slices

Day 17

Breakfast: Chia seed pudding with mixed berries

Lunch: Grilled chicken and vegetable skewers with a side of quinoa

Dinner: Beef and vegetable stir-fry with a side of brown rice

Snack: Celery sticks with almond butter

Day 18

Breakfast: Greek yogurt with a drizzle of honey and fresh fruit

Lunch: Quinoa salad with black beans, corn, and avocado

Dinner: Baked cod with roasted Brussels sprouts and sweet potatoes

Snack: A handful of walnuts

Day 19

Breakfast: Smoothie with kale, banana, and protein powder

Lunch: Turkey and spinach salad with balsamic vinaigrette

Dinner: Grilled shrimp with a side of mixed vegetables and brown rice

Snack: Greek yogurt with a sprinkle of chia seeds

Day 20

Breakfast: Overnight oats with chia seeds, almond milk, and fresh berries

Lunch: Chicken and vegetable soup with a side of whole-grain crackers

Dinner: Grilled pork chops with a side of mashed sweet potatoes and sautéed kale

Snack: Fresh orange slices

Day 21

Breakfast: Avocado and egg on whole-grain toast

Lunch: Quinoa and chickpea salad with mixed greens and a lemon dressing

Dinner: Baked salmon with roasted carrots and green beans

Snack: Cottage cheese with pineapple chunks

Week 4

Day 22

Breakfast: Smoothie bowl with spinach, berries, and granola

Lunch: Lentil and vegetable stew with a side salad

Dinner: Chicken breast with a side of quinoa and steamed broccoli

Snack: Handful of almonds

Day 23

Breakfast: Greek yogurt with chia seeds and fresh fruit

Lunch: Turkey wrap with avocado and mixed greens

Dinner: Grilled tilapia with roasted sweet potatoes and sautéed spinach

Snack: Sliced bell peppers with guacamole

Day 24

Breakfast: Scrambled eggs with mushrooms and onions

Lunch: Quinoa and black bean salad with bell peppers and lime dressing

Dinner: Baked chicken thighs with a side of roasted Brussels sprouts and brown rice

Snack: Fresh apple slices with almond butter

Day 25

Breakfast: Overnight chia pudding with almond milk and fresh berries

Lunch: Grilled chicken salad with mixed greens and a vinaigrette

Dinner: Beef and vegetable stir-fry with cauliflower rice

Snack: Fresh berries

Day 26

Breakfast: Smoothie with spinach, banana, and protein powder

Lunch: Chickpea and vegetable curry with a side of quinoa

Dinner: Grilled shrimp with a side of roasted sweet potatoes and green beans

Snack: Celery sticks with almond butter

Day 27

Breakfast: Chia seed pudding topped with kiwi and coconut flakes

Lunch: Tuna salad with mixed greens and a side of whole-grain crackers

Dinner: Baked haddock with a side of roasted carrots and wild rice

Snack: Handful of walnuts

Day 28

Breakfast: Avocado toast on whole-grain bread with a poached egg

Lunch: Spinach and feta-stuffed chicken breast with a side salad

Dinner: Stuffed bell peppers with ground turkey and cauliflower rice

Snack: Greek yogurt with honey

Day 29

Breakfast: Smoothie bowl with kale, frozen berries, and granola

Lunch: Turkey and avocado lettuce wraps with a side of mixed veggies

Dinner: Baked salmon with quinoa and steamed broccoli

Snack: Sliced cucumber with hummus

Day 30

Breakfast: Scrambled eggs with spinach and a side of fresh fruit

Lunch: Quinoa salad with black beans, corn, and avocado

Dinner: Grilled pork chops with mashed sweet potatoes and sautéed kale

Snack: Cottage cheese with pineapple chunks

Leftovers Suggestions

To make the most of your meals, here's how you can creatively use leftovers:

Day 2 Dinner Leftovers: Use the turkey and vegetable stir-fry as a filling for wraps or as a topping for salads.

Day 5 Lunch Leftovers: The chickpea and vegetable curry can be used as a topping for quinoa or a filling for a wrap.

Day 8 Lunch Leftovers: Chicken and vegetable soup can be enjoyed as a hearty broth or served with a side salad.

Day 13 Dinner Leftovers: Beef fajitas can be used in wraps or as a topping for salads.

Day 17 Dinner Leftovers: Stuffed zucchini boats can be repurposed as a filling for lettuce wraps or served with a side of quinoa.

Day 20 Dinner Leftovers: Grilled pork chops can be sliced and added to salads or used in sandwiches.

This meal plan aims to provide variety while supporting adrenal health through balanced meals and smart use of leftovers. Enjoy the journey to better health with each nourishing meal!

Chapter Six

Recipes for Adrenal Healing

Here are some breakfast recipes designed for the Adrenal Reset Diet. Each recipe includes detailed ingredients, step-by-step instructions, and a description of the colors, textures, smells, and tastes of the dishes.

Spinach and Mushroom Egg Muffins

Ingredients:

6 large eggs

1 cup fresh spinach, chopped

1/2 cup mushrooms, diced

1/4 cup feta cheese, crumbled

1/4 cup milk (any kind)

Salt and pepper to taste

Olive oil spray

Instructions:

Preheat your oven to 375°F (190°C) and lightly spray a muffin tin with olive oil.

Sauté the mushrooms in a non-stick pan over medium heat until they are tender and slightly golden, about 5 minutes. Add the chopped spinach and cook until wilted, about 2 minutes.

Whisk the eggs and milk together in a bowl. Season with salt and pepper.

Combine the sautéed mushrooms and spinach with the egg mixture. Stir in the crumbled feta cheese.

Pour the mixture evenly into the muffin tin cups, filling each about 3/4 full.

Bake for 20-25 minutes, or until the egg muffins are set and lightly browned on top.

Cool slightly before removing from the tin.

Description: The egg muffins emerge golden brown on the edges, with a vibrant green hue from the spinach and speckles of white feta cheese. The texture is fluffy and light, with a rich, savory aroma from the sautéed mushrooms. The taste is a delightful blend of creamy feta, earthy mushrooms, and fresh spinach, making each bite satisfying and nutritious.

Berry Chia Pudding

Ingredients:

1/4 cup chia seeds

1 cup unsweetened almond milk

1 tablespoon maple syrup or honey

1/2 teaspoon vanilla extract

1/2 cup mixed berries (blueberries, strawberries, raspberries)

Instructions:

Mix the chia seeds, almond milk, maple syrup, and vanilla extract in a bowl. Stir well.

Refrigerate the mixture for at least 4 hours, or overnight, allowing the chia seeds to absorb the liquid and thicken into a pudding-like consistency.

Top the chia pudding with mixed berries before serving.

Description: The chia pudding has a creamy, pudding-like texture with a hint of sweetness. It is speckled with plump, juicy berries that burst with color—red strawberries, deep blue blueberries, and vibrant raspberries. The aroma is subtle, with a hint of vanilla and the fresh scent of berries. The taste is a balanced mix of sweet and tangy, with a smooth and satisfying mouthfeel.

Avocado and Tomato Smoothie

Ingredients:

1 ripe avocado

1 large tomato, peeled and chopped

1/2 cucumber, peeled and chopped

1 cup spinach

1 tablespoon lime juice

Salt and pepper to taste

1 cup water or coconut water

Instructions:

Combine the avocado, tomato, cucumber, spinach, lime juice, and water in a blender.

Blend until smooth and creamy.

Season with salt and pepper to taste.

Description: The smoothie is a vibrant green color with flecks of red and orange from the tomato. It has a creamy texture, smooth and refreshing on the palate. The smell is light and herbal with a hint of citrus from the lime juice. The taste is a refreshing blend of creamy avocado and tangy tomato, with a hint of lime to brighten the flavors.

Sweet Potato Hash with Eggs

Ingredients:

1 large sweet potato, peeled and diced

1 red bell pepper, diced

1 small onion, chopped

2 cloves garlic, minced

2 eggs

1 tablespoon olive oil

Salt and pepper to taste

Fresh parsley, chopped (optional)

Instructions:

Heat olive oil in a skillet over medium heat.

Add the diced sweet potato and cook until tender and lightly caramelized, about 10 minutes.

Stir in the bell pepper, onion, and garlic. Cook until vegetables are tender, about 5 minutes.

Season with salt and pepper.

Create two wells in the hash and crack an egg into each well.

Cover and cook until the eggs are done to your liking, about 5-7 minutes for sunny-side up.

Garnish with fresh parsley if desired.

Description: The sweet potato hash is colorful with orange sweet potatoes, red bell peppers, and green parsley. The texture is a delightful mix of crispy edges and tender centers. The aroma is hearty and savory, with hints of garlic and caramelized sweet potatoes. The taste combines the natural sweetness of sweet potatoes with savory eggs and aromatic vegetables.

Greek Yogurt with Fresh Fruit and Nuts

Ingredients:

1 cup Greek yogurt

1/2 cup mixed fresh fruit (berries, apple slices, or banana)

2 tablespoons mixed nuts (almonds, walnuts, or pecans)

1 tablespoon honey or maple syrup (optional)

Instructions:

Spoon the Greek yogurt into a bowl.

Top with fresh fruit and mixed nuts.

Drizzle with honey or maple syrup if desired.

Description: The Greek yogurt is creamy and thick, topped with a colorful array of fresh fruit and crunchy nuts. The texture is a pleasing combination of smooth yogurt and crunchy nuts. The aroma is mildly sweet with hints of honey and fresh fruit. The taste is creamy and tangy from the yogurt, complemented by the natural sweetness of the fruit and the crunch of the nuts.

Almond Flour Pancakes

Ingredients:

1 cup almond flour

2 large eggs

1/4 cup almond milk

1 tablespoon honey or maple syrup

1/2 teaspoon baking powder

1/2 teaspoon vanilla extract

Butter or coconut oil for cooking

Instructions:

Mix almond flour, eggs, almond milk, honey, baking powder, and vanilla extract in a bowl until smooth.

100 | Adrenal Reset Diet for Beginners

Heat a skillet over medium heat and add a small amount of butter or coconut oil.

Pour batter into the skillet to form pancakes, cooking until bubbles form on the surface. Flip and cook until golden brown.

Serve with fresh fruit or a drizzle of honey.

Description: The almond flour pancakes have a golden-brown color with a fluffy, slightly dense texture. The aroma is warm and nutty with a hint of vanilla. The taste is subtly sweet and nutty, with a satisfying crumbly texture that pairs well with the fresh fruit.

Savory Quinoa Breakfast Bowl

Ingredients:

1/2 cup quinoa, rinsed

1 cup water or vegetable broth

1/2 cup cherry tomatoes, halved

1/2 avocado, sliced

1/4 cup crumbled feta cheese

1 tablespoon olive oil

Salt and pepper to taste

Instructions:

Bring water or broth to a boil in a small pot. Add quinoa, reduce heat, and simmer for 15 minutes or until water is absorbed.

Fluff the quinoa with a fork and transfer to a bowl.

Top with cherry tomatoes, avocado slices, and crumbled feta cheese.

Drizzle with olive oil and season with salt and pepper.

Description: The breakfast bowl is visually appealing with vibrant red tomatoes, green avocado, and white feta cheese atop golden quinoa. The texture is a mix of fluffy quinoa, creamy avocado, and juicy tomatoes. The aroma is fresh and savory with hints of feta.

The taste is a delightful combination of creamy avocado, tangy feta, and sweet tomatoes.

Banana and Almond Butter Smoothie

Ingredients:

1 ripe banana

2 tablespoons almond butter

1 cup unsweetened almond milk

1/2 teaspoon cinnamon

Ice cubes (optional)

Instructions:

Combine the banana, almond butter, almond milk, and cinnamon in a blender.

Blend until smooth and creamy. Add ice cubes if desired for a colder smoothie.

Pour into a glass and enjoy.

Description: The smoothie is creamy and light beige with a thick, velvety texture. The aroma is warm and nutty with a hint of cinnamon. The taste is sweet and nutty from the banana and almond butter, with a comforting warmth from the cinnamon.

Cottage Cheese with Pineapple and Chia Seeds

Ingredients:

1 cup cottage cheese

1/2 cup fresh pineapple chunks

1 tablespoon chia seeds

1 tablespoon honey (optional)

Instructions:

Combine the cottage cheese and pineapple chunks in a bowl.

Stir in chia seeds and honey if using.

Serve immediately or chill for later.

Description: The cottage cheese is creamy and white, mixed with vibrant yellow pineapple chunks. The chia seeds add a slight crunch. The texture is a pleasing mix of smooth and chunky. The aroma is fresh and tropical. The taste combines the tangy

Scrambled Eggs with Spinach and Avocado

Ingredients:

2 large eggs

1 cup fresh spinach, chopped

1/2 avocado, sliced

1 tablespoon olive oil

Salt and pepper to taste

Fresh parsley (optional)

Instructions:

Heat the olive oil in a skillet over medium heat.

105 | Adrenal Reset Diet for Beginners

Add the chopped spinach to the skillet and sauté for about 2-3 minutes until wilted.

Crack the eggs into a bowl, whisk them, and season with salt and pepper.

Pour the eggs into the skillet with the spinach, scrambling them gently until they're fully cooked but still fluffy.

Serve the scrambled eggs alongside fresh avocado slices, optionally garnishing with fresh parsley for added flavor and color.

Description: This dish presents a vibrant contrast with the golden-yellow scrambled eggs, speckled with bright green spinach, and creamy avocado slices on the side. The eggs are light and fluffy, while the sautéed spinach adds an earthy aroma and a subtle bite. The creamy texture of the avocado adds a rich, buttery taste that complements the savory eggs. The fresh parsley brings a touch of brightness to the dish both in taste and color.

Lunch Recipes

Here some Adrenal Reset Diet Lunch Recipes, complete with detailed ingredients, step-by-step instructions, and sensory descriptions to bring the dishes to life:

Quinoa and Avocado Salad

Ingredients:

1 cup cooked quinoa

1 ripe avocado, diced

1/2 cup cherry tomatoes, halved

1/4 cup red onion, finely chopped

2 tablespoons olive oil

1 tablespoon lemon juice

Salt and pepper to taste

Fresh parsley for garnish

Instructions:

Cook the quinoa according to package instructions. Let it cool.

In a large bowl, combine the quinoa, diced avocado, cherry tomatoes, and red onion.

Drizzle with olive oil and lemon juice, then season with salt and pepper.

Gently toss to combine, being careful not to mash the avocado.

Garnish with fresh parsley before serving.

Description: This salad is a riot of colors, from the fluffy white quinoa to the bright green avocado and juicy red cherry tomatoes. The quinoa offers a soft and slightly nutty texture, while the avocado adds creaminess. The lemon juice brings a fresh, tangy aroma, balancing the rich taste of the avocado. Each bite is light yet satisfying, with bursts of freshness from the parsley.

Grilled Chicken with Sweet Potato Mash

Ingredients:

1 boneless chicken breast

1 medium sweet potato

1 tablespoon olive oil

Salt and pepper to taste

1/2 teaspoon paprika

Fresh thyme for garnish

Instructions:

Season the chicken breast with olive oil, salt, pepper, and paprika.

Grill the chicken on medium heat for about 5-6 minutes on each side until fully cooked.

Peel and dice the sweet potato, then boil in salted water until tender, about 10-12 minutes.

Mash the sweet potato with a fork, seasoning with salt and pepper to taste.

Serve the grilled chicken over a bed of sweet potato mash and garnish with fresh thyme.

Description: The chicken has a golden, grilled exterior with a smoky aroma, contrasting beautifully with the velvety orange of the sweet potato mash. The texture of the mash is smooth and buttery, while the chicken is tender and juicy. The earthy scent of thyme ties the dish together, providing a warm, comforting flavor in every bite.

Lentil and Vegetable Stew

Ingredients:

1 cup green or brown lentils, rinsed

1 carrot, diced

1 zucchini, diced

1 onion, chopped

2 garlic cloves, minced

4 cups vegetable broth

1 tablespoon olive oil

Salt and pepper to taste

1 bay leaf

Fresh parsley for garnish

Instructions:

Heat olive oil in a large pot over medium heat. Add onion and garlic, sautéing until fragrant, about 3 minutes.

Add the diced carrot, zucchini, and lentils. Stir well.

Pour in the vegetable broth, add the bay leaf, and bring to a boil.

Reduce heat to a simmer, cooking for 25-30 minutes until lentils are tender.

Season with salt and pepper, remove the bay leaf, and garnish with fresh parsley.

Description: This stew has an inviting earthy aroma, with the rich, brown lentils contrasting against bright orange carrots and green zucchini. The broth is flavorful and hearty, with a slight chew from the lentils. The dish is rustic and comforting, with a savory depth from the bay leaf and garlic.

Zucchini Noodles with Pesto and Cherry Tomatoes

Ingredients:

2 medium zucchinis, spiralized

1/2 cup cherry tomatoes, halved

1/4 cup pesto (store-bought or homemade)

1 tablespoon olive oil

Salt and pepper to taste

Fresh basil for garnish

Instructions:

Heat olive oil in a pan over medium heat. Add the zucchini noodles and sauté for 2-3 minutes until tender but not mushy.

Toss the zucchini noodles with pesto, making sure they are evenly coated.

Add the cherry tomatoes and sauté for another 1-2 minutes until they soften slightly.

Season with salt and pepper, then garnish with fresh basil before serving.

Description: The vibrant green of the zucchini noodles is enhanced by the deep, herbal green of the pesto. Bright red cherry tomatoes add a pop of color. The texture is light and crisp from the zucchini, while the pesto provides a rich, garlicky aroma. The flavors are fresh and vibrant, with a slightly nutty taste from the pesto and a burst of sweetness from the tomatoes.

Chickpea and Spinach Stir-Fry

Ingredients:

1 can chickpeas, drained and rinsed

2 cups fresh spinach

1 small onion, sliced

2 garlic cloves, minced

1 tablespoon olive oil

1 teaspoon cumin

Salt and pepper to taste

Fresh lemon wedges for serving

Instructions:

Heat olive oil in a skillet over medium heat. Add the onion and garlic, sautéing until translucent, about 3 minutes.

Add the chickpeas and cumin, stirring well. Cook for another 5 minutes until the chickpeas are slightly crispy.

Toss in the spinach and cook for another 2-3 minutes until wilted.

Season with salt and pepper, and serve with a squeeze of fresh lemon juice.

Description: The golden-brown chickpeas are crisp on the outside, blending beautifully with the wilted dark green spinach. The aroma is warm and inviting, with earthy cumin and bright citrus from the lemon. The texture is a contrast of crispy chickpeas and tender spinach, with the tang of lemon adding a refreshing finish to the dish.

Turkey Lettuce Wraps

Ingredients:

1/2 pound ground turkey

1 tablespoon olive oil

1 small onion, chopped

1 carrot, grated

1 tablespoon soy sauce or tamari

1 teaspoon ginger, minced

8 large lettuce leaves

Sesame seeds for garnish

Instructions:

Heat olive oil in a skillet over medium heat. Add the onion and ginger, sautéing for 2-3 minutes until fragrant.

Add the ground turkey and cook until browned, about 5-7 minutes.

Stir in the grated carrot and soy sauce, cooking for another 2 minutes until the carrot is tender.

Spoon the turkey mixture into lettuce leaves and garnish with sesame seeds.

Description: The vibrant green lettuce wraps cradle the savory, golden-brown turkey filling. The turkey is juicy and tender, with a subtle warmth from the ginger. The crisp lettuce adds a fresh, crunchy contrast to the soft turkey filling, making each bite a perfect balance of textures.

Mediterranean Tuna Salad

Ingredients:

1 can tuna, drained

1/2 cup cucumber, diced

1/2 cup cherry tomatoes, halved

1/4 cup red onion, finely chopped

1/4 cup kalamata olives, sliced

2 tablespoons olive oil

1 tablespoon lemon juice

Salt and pepper to taste

Fresh parsley for garnish

Instructions:

In a bowl, combine tuna, cucumber, cherry tomatoes, red onion, and olives.

117 | Adrenal Reset Diet for Beginners

Drizzle with olive oil and lemon juice, then season with salt and pepper.

Gently toss and garnish with fresh parsley before serving.

Description: The salad is a medley of Mediterranean colors, from the red cherry tomatoes to the green cucumbers and black olives. The texture is light yet crunchy, with the tuna providing a hearty, flaky base. The smell is fresh with citrusy lemon, and the taste is bright, tangy, and slightly salty from the olives, making it refreshing and filling.

Grilled Salmon with Asparagus

Ingredients:

1 salmon fillet

1 bunch asparagus, trimmed

1 tablespoon olive oil

Salt and pepper to taste

Lemon wedges for serving

Instructions:

Heat a grill pan over medium heat. Brush the salmon fillet and asparagus with olive oil, then season with salt and pepper.

Grill the salmon for 4-5 minutes on each side until the flesh is opaque and flaky.

Grill the asparagus for 3-4 minutes until tender with slight grill marks.

Serve the salmon and asparagus with fresh lemon wedges.

Description: The salmon has a beautiful golden sear, with tender flakes of pink flesh underneath. The asparagus is bright green with charred edges, adding a slight smokiness. The aroma is fresh and lemony, with a hint of the sea. The taste is delicate and buttery from the salmon, with the crisp asparagus providing a perfect textural contrast.

119 | Adrenal Reset Diet for Beginners

Baked Falafel with Tahini Sauce

Ingredients:

1 can chickpeas, drained

1/4 cup fresh parsley

1/4 cup fresh cilantro

1 small onion, chopped

2 garlic cloves, minced

2 tablespoons flour

1 teaspoon cumin

Salt and pepper to taste

1 tablespoon olive oil

Tahini sauce for serving

Instructions:

Preheat the oven to 375°F (190°C).

In a food processor, combine chickpeas, parsley, cilantro, onion, garlic, flour, cumin, salt, and pepper. Pulse until the mixture forms a coarse dough.

Shape the mixture into small patties and place on a baking sheet lined with parchment paper.

Brush with olive oil and bake for 25-30 minutes until golden brown, flipping halfway through.

Serve with tahini sauce.

Description: The falafel patties are golden and crispy on the outside, with a soft, herb-packed interior. The smell of fresh parsley and cilantro fills the air as they bake. Each bite is crunchy, savory, and full of aromatic spices, complemented by the creamy, nutty flavor of the tahini sauce.

Spinach and Feta Stuffed Bell Peppers

Ingredients:

2 large bell peppers, halved and seeds removed

1 cup fresh spinach, chopped

1/2 cup feta cheese, crumbled

1 small onion, chopped

2 garlic cloves, minced

1 tablespoon olive oil

Salt and pepper to taste

Instructions:

Preheat the oven to 375°F (190°C).

In a skillet, heat olive oil and sauté onion and garlic until fragrant, about 3 minutes.

Add the chopped spinach and cook until wilted.

Remove from heat and stir in the crumbled feta cheese. Season with salt and pepper.

Stuff the bell pepper halves with the spinach-feta mixture.

Bake for 20-25 minutes until the peppers are tender.

Description: The vibrant colors of the bell peppers, with their bright red, yellow, or green skin, contrast beautifully with the creamy white feta and deep green spinach filling. The peppers are tender, slightly sweet, and filled with the savory, tangy taste of feta cheese. The aroma is warm and inviting, with hints of garlic and onion.

Dinner Recipes

Here are some Adrenal Reset Diet Dinner Recipes that are flavorful, colorful, and easy to prepare, complete with detailed instructions and sensory descriptions:

Lemon Herb Grilled Chicken with Roasted Vegetables

Ingredients:

2 boneless chicken breasts

1 tablespoon olive oil

1 tablespoon lemon juice

1 teaspoon dried thyme

1 teaspoon dried rosemary

Salt and pepper to taste

1 zucchini, sliced

1 bell pepper, sliced

1 red onion, sliced

Instructions:

Marinate the chicken breasts in olive oil, lemon juice, thyme, rosemary, salt, and pepper for 30 minutes.

Preheat the grill to medium heat. Grill the chicken for 6-7 minutes on each side until cooked through.

Roast the vegetables in the oven at 400°F (200°C) for 20-25 minutes, drizzled with olive oil, salt, and pepper.

Serve the grilled chicken alongside the roasted vegetables.

Description: The chicken is golden with grill marks, bursting with citrusy and herbal aromas. The roasted vegetables are vibrant – green zucchini, red peppers, and purple onion – with slightly charred edges that add a smoky depth. The chicken is tender and juicy, and the vegetables have a slight crunch with a hint of sweetness from roasting.

Baked Salmon with Garlic and Dill

Ingredients:

2 salmon fillets

1 tablespoon olive oil

2 garlic cloves, minced

125 | Adrenal Reset Diet for Beginners

1 tablespoon fresh dill, chopped

1 lemon, sliced

Salt and pepper to taste

Instructions:

Preheat the oven to 375°F (190°C).

Place the salmon fillets on a baking sheet lined with parchment paper. Drizzle with olive oil, sprinkle with minced garlic, fresh dill, salt, and pepper.

Top each fillet with lemon slices.

Bake for 12-15 minutes until the salmon is flaky and opaque.

Serve with a fresh salad or steamed vegetables.

Description: The salmon emerges from the oven with a light pink color, topped with golden lemon slices. The scent of garlic and fresh dill fills the air. The texture is tender and flaky, with a delicate, buttery taste balanced by the zesty lemon and aromatic herbs.

Quinoa-Stuffed Bell Peppers

Ingredients:

4 large bell peppers, tops cut off and seeds removed

1 cup cooked quinoa

1/2 cup black beans, drained and rinsed

1/2 cup corn kernels

1/4 cup chopped tomatoes

1 teaspoon cumin

1 tablespoon olive oil

Salt and pepper to taste

Fresh cilantro for garnish

Instructions:

Preheat the oven to 375°F (190°C).

In a bowl, mix the cooked quinoa, black beans, corn, tomatoes, olive oil, cumin, salt, and pepper.

Stuff the bell peppers with the quinoa mixture.

Bake the stuffed peppers for 25-30 minutes until the peppers are tender.

Garnish with fresh cilantro before serving.

Description: The bell peppers retain their bright colors – red, yellow, or orange – while becoming tender and slightly charred at the edges. The stuffing is a colorful blend of quinoa, black beans, and corn, with a savory, earthy aroma from the cumin. Each bite offers a hearty, protein-packed filling inside the sweet, roasted pepper.

Shrimp Stir-Fry with Broccoli and Carrots

Ingredients:

1/2 pound shrimp, peeled and deveined

2 cups broccoli florets

1 carrot, thinly sliced

1 tablespoon soy sauce or tamari

1 tablespoon olive oil

2 garlic cloves, minced

1 teaspoon ginger, minced

Instructions:

Heat olive oil in a large pan over medium heat. Add garlic and ginger, sautéing until fragrant.

Add the shrimp and cook for 3-4 minutes until they turn pink.

Remove the shrimp from the pan and set aside.

Add the broccoli and carrots to the pan, sautéing for 5-7 minutes until tender.

Return the shrimp to the pan, drizzle with soy sauce, and toss everything together.

Serve hot.

129 | Adrenal Reset Diet for Beginners

Description: The shrimp turns a vibrant pink, while the broccoli remains a bright, crunchy green. The carrots add a touch of orange to the dish. The aroma is savory with hints of garlic and ginger, and the soy sauce adds a salty, umami depth. The shrimp are tender and juicy, while the vegetables have a perfect bite.

Zucchini Lasagna

Ingredients:

2 large zucchinis, sliced lengthwise into thin strips

1/2 pound ground turkey or beef

1 cup marinara sauce

1/2 cup ricotta cheese

1/4 cup mozzarella cheese, shredded

1/4 cup Parmesan cheese, grated

1 teaspoon oregano

Salt and pepper to taste

Instructions:

Preheat the oven to 375°F (190°C).

Cook the ground turkey in a skillet over medium heat, seasoning with oregano, salt, and pepper. Stir in the marinara sauce.

Layer the zucchini strips in a baking dish, alternating with the meat sauce and dollops of ricotta cheese.

Top with mozzarella and Parmesan cheese.

Bake for 30-35 minutes until the cheese is bubbly and golden.

Let rest for 5 minutes before serving.

Description: The lasagna has a golden-brown crust of melted cheese, with layers of tender zucchini and hearty meat sauce peeking through. The smell of oregano and marinara sauce wafts through the kitchen. The texture is creamy and cheesy, with a satisfying richness from the ricotta and turkey, while the zucchini adds a lightness to each bite.

Chicken and Vegetable Skewers

Ingredients:

2 boneless chicken breasts, cubed

1 zucchini, sliced into rounds

1 bell pepper, cubed

1 red onion, cubed

2 tablespoons olive oil

1 tablespoon lemon juice

1 teaspoon paprika

Salt and pepper to taste

Instructions:

Preheat the grill or oven to 375°F (190°C).

Marinate the chicken and vegetables in olive oil, lemon juice, paprika, salt, and pepper for 20 minutes.

Thread the chicken and vegetables onto skewers.

Grill or bake for 15-20 minutes, turning occasionally, until the chicken is fully cooked.

Serve with a side of quinoa or a fresh salad.

Description: The skewers are visually vibrant, with the golden-brown chicken cubes interspersed with the brightly colored vegetables – green zucchini, red bell pepper, and purple onion. The grilled aroma is smoky and savory, and the chicken is juicy and tender, with a slight char from the grill. The vegetables are slightly crisp and bursting with fresh flavor.

Turkey and Spinach Meatballs

Ingredients:

133 | Adrenal Reset Diet for Beginners

1/2 pound ground turkey

1 cup fresh spinach, chopped

1/4 cup almond flour

1 egg

2 garlic cloves, minced

1 teaspoon Italian seasoning

Salt and pepper to taste

Instructions:

Preheat the oven to 375°F (190°C).

In a bowl, mix together the ground turkey, chopped spinach, almond flour, egg, garlic, Italian seasoning, salt, and pepper.

Shape the mixture into small meatballs and place them on a baking sheet.

Bake for 20-25 minutes until golden brown and fully cooked.

Serve with a side of marinara sauce or steamed vegetables.

Description: The meatballs are golden and slightly crisp on the outside, with vibrant green flecks of spinach throughout. The aroma of garlic and Italian herbs fills the air as they bake. Inside, they are moist and tender, with the spinach adding a fresh, earthy note. Each bite is savory and perfectly seasoned.

Eggplant and Chickpea Stew

Ingredients:

1 large eggplant, cubed

1 can chickpeas, drained and rinsed

1 can diced tomatoes

1 onion, chopped

2 garlic cloves, minced

1 tablespoon olive oil

1 teaspoon cumin

Salt and pepper to taste

135 | Adrenal Reset Diet for Beginners

Fresh parsley for garnish

Instructions:

Heat olive oil in a large pot over medium heat. Add the onion and garlic, sautéing until fragrant.

Add the cubed eggplant and cook for 5-7 minutes until softened.

Stir in the chickpeas, diced tomatoes, cumin, salt, and pepper.

Simmer for 20-25 minutes, stirring occasionally.

Garnish with fresh parsley before serving.

Description: The stew is a hearty, rich dish, with the soft, golden-brown eggplant absorbing the flavors of the tomatoes and spices. The chickpeas add a satisfying bite. The smell of cumin fills the air, adding a warm, slightly earthy scent. The stew is thick and comforting, with a balance of tangy tomatoes and creamy chickpeas.

Grilled Lemon and Herb Shrimp

Ingredients:

1/2 pound large shrimp, peeled and deveined

1 tablespoon olive oil

1 tablespoon lemon juice

1 teaspoon dried oregano

Salt and pepper to taste

Instructions:

Preheat the grill or a grill pan to medium heat.

Marinate the shrimp in olive oil, lemon juice, oregano, salt, and pepper for 15 minutes.

Grill the shrimp for 2-3 minutes on each side until they are pink and slightly charred.

Serve with a side of grilled vegetables or salad.

Description: The shrimp are vibrant pink with char marks from the grill, infused with the zesty tang of lemon and the fresh, herbal notes of oregano. They are juicy and slightly smoky, with a burst of citrus flavor in every bite. The aroma is mouthwatering, with the shrimp smelling of the sea and herbs.

Baked Cod with Garlic and Thyme

Ingredients:

2 cod fillets

1 tablespoon olive oil

2 garlic cloves, minced

1 teaspoon fresh thyme leaves

Salt and pepper to taste

Lemon wedges for serving

Instructions:

Preheat the oven to 375°F (190°C).

Place the cod fillets on a baking sheet and drizzle with olive oil.

Sprinkle with minced garlic, fresh thyme, salt, and pepper.

Bake for 10-12 minutes until the fish is flaky and opaque.

Serve with lemon wedges and a side of steamed vegetables.

Description: The cod fillets are a pristine white, flaking easily with a fork, and topped with golden flecks of garlic and fresh thyme. The aroma is fresh and fragrant, with the thyme adding an earthy, floral scent. The fish is light and buttery, with a mild flavor that pairs perfectly with the zesty lemon juice.

Snacks and Dessert

Here are some Adrenal Reset Diet Snacks and Dessert Recipes with detailed descriptions of ingredients, steps, and the sensory experience:

Almond Butter Energy Balls

Ingredients:

1 cup rolled oats

1/2 cup almond butter

1/4 cup honey or maple syrup

1/4 cup flaxseeds

1/4 cup dark chocolate chips

1 teaspoon vanilla extract

Instructions:

In a bowl, mix the oats, almond butter, honey, flaxseeds, dark chocolate chips, and vanilla extract.

Roll the mixture into small balls using your hands.

Place the energy balls on a baking sheet and refrigerate for 30 minutes to set.

Store in an airtight container in the fridge.

Description: These energy balls are chewy and slightly crunchy, with the deep, nutty flavor of almond butter. The oats provide a soft base, while the dark chocolate chips add a hint of sweetness. The flaxseeds give the snack a light crunch, and the subtle sweetness of honey ties it all together. Their rich aroma is a mix of nutty and sweet.

Coconut Chia Pudding

Ingredients:

1/4 cup chia seeds

1 cup coconut milk

1 tablespoon maple syrup

1/2 teaspoon vanilla extract

Fresh berries for topping

141 | Adrenal Reset Diet for Beginners

Instructions:

In a bowl, combine chia seeds, coconut milk, maple syrup, and vanilla extract.

Stir well and let sit for 5 minutes, then stir again to prevent clumping.

Refrigerate for 2 hours or overnight until the pudding thickens.

Top with fresh berries before serving.

Description: The chia pudding is smooth and creamy with a rich coconut flavor. The tiny chia seeds add a fun, slightly crunchy texture. The pudding is topped with bright, juicy berries that burst with sweetness and color, providing a perfect balance to the silky base. The smell is light and tropical with a hint of vanilla.

Apple Slices with Almond Butter and Cinnamon

Ingredients:

1 apple, sliced

2 tablespoons almond butter

1/2 teaspoon cinnamon

A sprinkle of chia seeds (optional)

Instructions:

Arrange the apple slices on a plate.

Spread almond butter over each slice.

Sprinkle with cinnamon and chia seeds.

Description: The apple slices are crisp and juicy, with a sweet-tart flavor that complements the smooth, rich almond butter. The cinnamon adds a warm, spicy note, while the chia seeds offer a slight crunch. The colors are simple but inviting – light green or red apples with the golden almond butter and a dusting of cinnamon.

Dark Chocolate-Covered Strawberries

Ingredients:

1 cup fresh strawberries

1/2 cup dark chocolate, melted

Instructions:

Wash and dry the strawberries thoroughly.

Melt the dark chocolate in a microwave or double boiler.

Dip each strawberry into the melted chocolate, covering about two-thirds of the fruit.

Place on a baking sheet lined with parchment paper and refrigerate for 30 minutes until the chocolate hardens.

Description: These strawberries are visually stunning, with the rich, dark chocolate providing a glossy coat over the bright red fruit. The contrast between the snap of the firm chocolate and the juicy, sweet strawberry inside is divine. The smell is a decadent mix of rich cocoa and fresh, fruity aromas.

Baked Sweet Potato Chips

Ingredients:

2 medium sweet potatoes, thinly sliced

1 tablespoon olive oil

Salt to taste

A pinch of paprika (optional)

Instructions:

Preheat the oven to 375°F (190°C).

Toss the sweet potato slices with olive oil, salt, and paprika.

Arrange the slices in a single layer on a baking sheet.

Bake for 15-20 minutes, flipping halfway through, until crispy.

145 | Adrenal Reset Diet for Beginners

Description: The chips are a golden orange with crispy edges and a slight chew in the center. They have a savory, slightly sweet flavor with a hint of smokiness from the paprika. The smell of roasting sweet potatoes fills the kitchen, creating a warm and inviting atmosphere.

Avocado Chocolate Mousse

Ingredients:

2 ripe avocados

1/4 cup cocoa powder

1/4 cup maple syrup

1/2 teaspoon vanilla extract

A pinch of sea salt

Instructions:

Blend the avocados, cocoa powder, maple syrup, vanilla extract, and sea salt until smooth and creamy.

Chill in the fridge for 30 minutes before serving.

Garnish with fresh berries or a sprinkle of cocoa nibs.

Description: This mousse is silky and decadent, with a deep chocolate flavor balanced by the creamy avocado base. It has a velvety texture that melts in your mouth, and the richness of the cocoa is complemented by the subtle sweetness of the maple syrup. The dark color and creamy texture make it look indulgent, but it's surprisingly light and healthy.

Cinnamon-Spiced Roasted Almonds

Ingredients:

1 cup raw almonds

1 tablespoon coconut oil

1 tablespoon honey

147 | Adrenal Reset Diet for Beginners

1 teaspoon cinnamon

A pinch of sea salt

Instructions:

Preheat the oven to 350°F (175°C).

Melt the coconut oil and honey together in a small saucepan.

Toss the almonds with the coconut oil mixture, cinnamon, and salt.

Spread the almonds on a baking sheet and roast for 10-12 minutes, stirring halfway through.

Description: These roasted almonds are golden brown and slightly shiny from the coconut oil. They have a satisfying crunch, with a warm, sweet-spicy flavor from the cinnamon and honey. The aroma of cinnamon fills the room as they roast, creating a cozy, autumn-like atmosphere.

Cucumber and Hummus Bites

Ingredients:

1 cucumber, sliced into rounds

1/2 cup hummus

Paprika for garnish

Fresh parsley for garnish

Instructions:

Place a dollop of hummus on each cucumber round.

Sprinkle with paprika and garnish with fresh parsley.

Description: These bites are refreshing and light, with the cool crunch of cucumber paired with the creamy, savory hummus. The paprika adds a pop of color and a subtle smoky flavor, while the parsley provides a fresh, herby aroma. Each bite is crisp, smooth, and bursting with flavor.

Berry and Almond Yogurt Parfait

Ingredients:

1 cup plain Greek yogurt

1/2 cup mixed berries (blueberries, raspberries, strawberries)

1 tablespoon slivered almonds

1 teaspoon honey (optional)

Instructions:

Layer the Greek yogurt and berries in a glass or bowl.

Top with slivered almonds and drizzle with honey if desired.

Description: The parfait is a colorful and visually appealing snack, with the bright reds and blues of the berries contrasting against the creamy white yogurt. The almonds add a crunch, and the honey brings a touch of sweetness. The yogurt is tangy and smooth, while the berries are juicy and fresh, creating a perfect balance of textures and flavors.

Pumpkin Seed Trail Mix

Ingredients:

1/2 cup raw pumpkin seeds

1/4 cup dried cranberries

1/4 cup dark chocolate chunks

1/4 cup almonds

A pinch of sea salt

Instructions:

Mix the pumpkin seeds, dried cranberries, dark chocolate chunks, almonds, and sea salt in a bowl.

Store in an airtight container for snacking.

Description: The trail mix is a delightful combination of textures and flavors, with the crunchy pumpkin seeds and almonds, the chewy sweetness of the dried cranberries, and the rich, bitter notes of dark chocolate. The sea salt enhances the flavors, making this snack satisfying and energizing. The colors range from the earthy green of pumpkin seeds to the deep reds of cranberries and the glossy brown of chocolate.

These snacks and desserts are designed to satisfy cravings while supporting adrenal health, providing a balance of nutrients with flavors that are both comforting and delicious.

Soup and Stew Recipes

Here are some delicious Adrenal Reset Diet Soup and Stew Recipes with detailed descriptions of ingredients, steps, and sensory experiences:

Creamy Butternut Squash Soup

Ingredients:

1 medium butternut squash, peeled and cubed

1 onion, chopped

2 garlic cloves, minced

1 tablespoon olive oil

4 cups vegetable broth

1/2 cup coconut milk

Salt and pepper to taste

Fresh thyme for garnish

Instructions:

Sauté the onion and garlic in olive oil until soft and fragrant.

Add the cubed butternut squash and sauté for 5 minutes.

Pour in the vegetable broth, bring to a boil, then simmer for 20 minutes until the squash is tender.

Blend the soup until smooth, stir in the coconut milk, and season with salt and pepper.

Garnish with fresh thyme and serve.

Description: The soup is a vibrant golden-orange, creamy and smooth with a silky texture. The natural sweetness of the butternut squash is balanced by the savory onion and garlic, while the coconut milk adds a touch of richness. The scent is warm and inviting, with a hint of fresh thyme.

Lentil and Spinach Stew

Ingredients:

1 cup green lentils

1 onion, chopped

2 carrots, chopped

2 garlic cloves, minced

4 cups vegetable broth

2 cups fresh spinach

1 teaspoon cumin

Salt and pepper to taste

Lemon wedges for serving

Instructions:

Sauté the onion, garlic, and carrots in a large pot until soft.

Add the lentils and cumin, stirring to coat the lentils in the spices.

Pour in the broth, bring to a boil, and then simmer for 25 minutes until the lentils are tender.

Stir in the spinach and cook until wilted.

Season with salt, pepper, and a squeeze of lemon before serving.

Description: This hearty stew has a rich, earthy aroma from the cumin and lentils. The lentils are soft and absorb the flavors of the broth, while the spinach adds a fresh green color and slight bitterness. The stew is thick and comforting, with a zesty finish from the lemon.

Chicken and Vegetable Soup

Ingredients:

1 boneless, skinless chicken breast

1 onion, chopped

2 carrots, chopped

2 celery stalks, chopped

1 zucchini, chopped

4 cups chicken broth

1 bay leaf

Fresh parsley for garnish

Salt and pepper to taste

Instructions:

In a large pot, sauté the onion, carrots, and celery until softened.

Add the chicken breast and bay leaf, then pour in the chicken broth.

Bring to a boil, then reduce heat and simmer for 20 minutes.

Remove the chicken, shred it, and return it to the pot along with the zucchini.

Cook for an additional 10 minutes and season with salt, pepper, and parsley.

Description: The soup is colorful and vibrant with chunks of tender chicken and a variety of vegetables. The broth is light and savory, with a slightly sweet aroma from the carrots. The flavors meld together, creating a comforting, nourishing dish with fresh parsley adding a burst of color and freshness.

Zucchini and Basil Soup

Ingredients:

157 | Adrenal Reset Diet for Beginners

4 medium zucchinis, sliced

1 onion, chopped

2 garlic cloves, minced

1 tablespoon olive oil

4 cups vegetable broth

1/4 cup fresh basil leaves

Salt and pepper to taste

Instructions:

Sauté the onion and garlic in olive oil until fragrant.

Add the zucchini slices and cook for 5 minutes.

Pour in the broth, bring to a boil, then simmer for 15 minutes.

Blend the soup until smooth and stir in the fresh basil.

Season with salt and pepper before serving.

Description: This soup is a vibrant green, with a fresh, herby aroma from the basil. The zucchini is light and smooth, blending into a creamy texture without dairy. The soup is refreshing, with the subtle sweetness of zucchini and the bright, peppery flavor of basil.

Sweet Potato and Kale Stew

Ingredients:

2 large sweet potatoes, peeled and cubed

1 onion, chopped

2 garlic cloves, minced

1 tablespoon olive oil

4 cups vegetable broth

2 cups chopped kale

1 teaspoon smoked paprika

Salt and pepper to taste

159 | Adrenal Reset Diet for Beginners

Instructions:

Sauté the onion and garlic in olive oil until soft.

Add the sweet potatoes and smoked paprika, stirring to combine.

Pour in the broth and simmer for 20 minutes until the sweet potatoes are tender.

Stir in the kale and cook for 5 minutes until wilted.

Season with salt and pepper before serving.

Description: The stew is a warm orange color from the sweet potatoes, with bright green kale adding contrast. The sweet potatoes are soft and slightly sweet, while the kale adds a slight bitterness and chewy texture. The smoked paprika gives the stew a deep, earthy aroma with a hint of spice.

Broccoli and Ginger Soup

Ingredients:

4 cups broccoli florets

1 onion, chopped

1 garlic clove, minced

1-inch piece fresh ginger, grated

1 tablespoon olive oil

4 cups vegetable broth

Salt and pepper to taste

Instructions:

Sauté the onion, garlic, and ginger in olive oil until fragrant.

Add the broccoli and cook for 5 minutes.

Pour in the broth, bring to a boil, then simmer for 15 minutes.

Blend the soup until smooth and season with salt and pepper.

Description: The soup is a deep, vibrant green with the fresh, zesty aroma of ginger. The broccoli provides a rich, earthy flavor, while the ginger adds warmth and spice. The texture is smooth and creamy, with a slightly peppery finish.

Carrot and Turmeric Soup

Ingredients:

6 large carrots, peeled and chopped

1 onion, chopped

2 garlic cloves, minced

1 tablespoon olive oil

1 teaspoon ground turmeric

4 cups vegetable broth

Salt and pepper to taste

Fresh cilantro for garnish

Instructions:

Sauté the onion, garlic, and turmeric in olive oil until fragrant.

Add the carrots and cook for 5 minutes.

Pour in the broth, bring to a boil, then simmer for 20 minutes.

Blend the soup until smooth and season with salt and pepper.

Garnish with fresh cilantro before serving.

Description: This soup has a bright, sunny orange hue with a rich, earthy aroma from the turmeric. The carrots are sweet and smooth, while the turmeric adds a subtle warmth. The fresh cilantro on top adds a burst of freshness, balancing the rich flavors.

Coconut Chicken Curry Soup

Ingredients:

1 boneless, skinless chicken breast, diced

1 onion, chopped

2 garlic cloves, minced

1 tablespoon curry powder

1 can coconut milk

4 cups chicken broth

1 cup spinach

Salt and pepper to taste

Instructions:

Sauté the onion, garlic, and curry powder in a large pot until fragrant.

Add the diced chicken and cook until browned.

Pour in the coconut milk and

chicken broth, and bring to a simmer for 10 minutes until the chicken is cooked through. Stir in the spinach and cook until wilted.

Season with salt and pepper before serving.

Description: This soup is creamy and golden, with the rich, warming scent of curry spices and coconut. The chicken is tender and juicy, and the spinach adds a burst of fresh green color and flavor. The broth is velvety with a subtle sweetness from the coconut milk, perfectly balanced by the aromatic curry spices.

White Bean and Rosemary Stew

Ingredients:

2 cans white beans, drained and rinsed

1 onion, chopped

2 garlic cloves, minced

1 tablespoon olive oil

4 cups vegetable broth

1 sprig fresh rosemary

Salt and pepper to taste

Lemon zest for garnish

Instructions:

165 | Adrenal Reset Diet for Beginners

Sauté the onion and garlic in olive oil until soft and fragrant.

Add the white beans and rosemary, stirring to coat the beans with the flavors.

Pour in the vegetable broth and simmer for 15 minutes.

Remove the rosemary sprig and season with salt, pepper, and a pinch of lemon zest.

Description: The stew is thick and hearty, with the white beans offering a creamy, melt-in-your-mouth texture. The rosemary adds a piney, herbaceous aroma that perfumes the entire dish. The broth is light but rich in flavor, and the lemon zest on top adds a bright, citrusy finish.

Spiced Red Lentil Soup

Ingredients:

1 cup red lentils

1 onion, chopped

2 garlic cloves, minced

1 tablespoon olive oil

1 teaspoon cumin

1/2 teaspoon ground coriander

4 cups vegetable broth

Juice of 1 lemon

Fresh cilantro for garnish

Salt and pepper to taste

Instructions:

Sauté the onion, garlic, cumin, and coriander in olive oil until fragrant.

Add the red lentils and stir to coat with the spices.

Pour in the vegetable broth and bring to a boil, then simmer for 15 minutes until the lentils are soft.

167 | Adrenal Reset Diet for Beginners

Stir in the lemon juice and season with salt and pepper.

Garnish with fresh cilantro before serving.

Description: This soup has a deep, golden-orange color, with a thick, creamy consistency. The red lentils absorb the warm, earthy spices, giving the soup a bold, comforting flavor. The fresh cilantro and lemon juice brighten the dish with a hint of freshness, while the cumin and coriander provide a subtle smoky undertone.

These Adrenal Reset Diet soup and stew recipes offer a wide variety of flavors, textures, and aromas, all designed to nourish the body and support adrenal health while providing a satisfying and delicious eating experience.

Lifestyle Tips for Adrenal Health

Maintaining adrenal health is crucial for overall well-being, particularly when dealing with chronic stress or adrenal fatigue.

Incorporating specific lifestyle changes can significantly enhance your adrenal function and help you feel more balanced and energized.

Here's a comprehensive guide to optimizing your lifestyle for better adrenal health:

1. Prioritize Sleep

Quality sleep is essential for adrenal health. Aim for 7-9 hours of uninterrupted sleep each night to allow your body to repair and rejuvenate. Establish a consistent sleep routine by going to bed and waking up at the same time every day. Create a restful environment by keeping your bedroom cool, dark, and quiet. Consider incorporating relaxation techniques such as deep breathing or meditation before bed to promote restful sleep.

2. Manage Stress Effectively

Chronic stress can deplete adrenal reserves and contribute to adrenal fatigue. Develop effective stress management strategies, including:

Mindfulness and Meditation: Practice mindfulness or meditation daily to calm the mind and reduce stress. Even just a few minutes each day can help lower cortisol levels and promote relaxation.

Deep Breathing Exercises: Engage in deep breathing exercises to activate the parasympathetic nervous system, which helps counteract stress responses.

Physical Activity: Regular exercise, particularly activities like yoga, tai chi, or walking, can help manage stress and improve mood.

3. Stay Hydrated

Proper hydration is vital for adrenal health. Drink plenty of water throughout the day to support overall bodily functions and maintain electrolyte balance. Dehydration can exacerbate feelings of fatigue and stress, so ensure you're consuming adequate fluids.

4. Balanced Nutrition

Beyond diet-specific recommendations, focus on a well-rounded nutrition plan that includes:

Nutrient-Dense Foods: Incorporate a variety of fruits, vegetables, lean proteins, and healthy fats to ensure you're getting essential vitamins and minerals.

Regular Meals: Eat balanced meals and snacks throughout the day to keep blood sugar levels stable and avoid energy crashes.

Reduce Caffeine and Sugar: Minimize caffeine and sugar intake, as they can stress the adrenal glands and contribute to adrenal fatigue.

5. Establish Healthy Boundaries

Setting boundaries is crucial for managing stress and protecting your adrenal health. Learn to say no to commitments that overwhelm you, and prioritize activities that bring you joy and relaxation. Balance work and personal life by scheduling regular breaks and downtime.

6. Practice Relaxation Techniques

Incorporate relaxation techniques into your daily routine to help manage stress:

Progressive Muscle Relaxation: Practice tensing and then relaxing different muscle groups to reduce physical tension.

Aromatherapy: Use essential oils like lavender or chamomile to create a calming atmosphere and enhance relaxation.

7. Engage in Positive Social Interactions

Surround yourself with supportive and positive individuals who uplift and encourage you. Meaningful social connections can help buffer against stress and improve overall emotional well-being. Make time for activities with friends and family that bring joy and fulfillment.

8. Seek Professional Support

If you're struggling with chronic stress or adrenal fatigue, consider seeking professional support from a healthcare provider or therapist. They can offer personalized guidance, therapeutic interventions, and help you develop a comprehensive plan for managing stress and supporting adrenal health.

By integrating these lifestyle tips into your daily routine, you can support your adrenal health, improve your overall well-being,

Conclusion

Embracing the Adrenal Reset Diet

As we reach the conclusion of the Adrenal Reset Diet for Beginners, it's essential to reflect on the journey you've embarked upon and the transformative potential this diet offers.

This book is designed to support your adrenal health by balancing hormones, stabilizing energy levels, and fostering overall wellness. By now, you should have a solid understanding of how the adrenal glands function, how stress impacts them, and how diet can play a pivotal role in their recovery.

The Power of Adrenal Health

The adrenal glands, though small, play a monumental role in regulating your body's response to stress, maintaining energy levels, and managing crucial hormones. The Adrenal Reset Diet aims to restore balance and function to these vital organs through thoughtful nutritional strategies.

By focusing on nutrient-dense foods, cycling carbs and proteins, and adhering to a diet that supports your body's natural rhythms, you empower your body to heal and thrive.

Diet as a Tool for Healing

Throughout this journey, you've learned how to harness the power of diet to support adrenal function. The structured meal plans, including breakfasts, lunches, dinners, snacks, and soups, provide a varied and nutritious foundation.

Each recipe is crafted to offer balanced macronutrients and essential vitamins and minerals, contributing to reduced stress and improved adrenal health. The emphasis on whole, unprocessed foods, combined with the strategic cycling of carbs and proteins, supports optimal energy levels and hormonal balance.

Holistic Approach to Wellness

While diet is a cornerstone of adrenal health, it is equally important to adopt a holistic approach to wellness. The lifestyle tips provided—such as prioritizing sleep, managing stress, staying hydrated, and fostering positive relationships—complement the dietary changes and create a comprehensive support system for your adrenals.

Embracing practices like mindfulness, proper time management, and relaxation techniques enhances your overall well-being and reinforces the positive impacts of the Adrenal Reset Diet.

Empowerment Through Knowledge

Knowledge is a powerful tool in managing your health. Understanding the science behind adrenal health, recognizing signs of adrenal fatigue, and learning how to adapt your lifestyle and diet accordingly equips you to make informed decisions.

This empowerment enables you to take control of your health and implement lasting changes that promote vitality and resilience.

Commitment to Your Health Journey

Embarking on the Adrenal Reset Diet is a commitment to your long-term health and well-being. It requires dedication, patience, and consistency.

The recipes and guidelines offered in this book are designed to provide structure and support, but remember that individual needs may vary. Listening to your body and making adjustments as needed will help you achieve the best results.

As you complete the Adrenal Reset Diet program, take time to reflect on your progress and celebrate your achievements. The benefits of a well-nourished body and balanced hormones will extend beyond this diet, impacting your overall quality of life. Continue to apply the principles learned, and embrace a lifestyle that supports sustained adrenal health.

In closing, the journey to better adrenal health is one of empowerment, self-discovery, and transformation. By integrating the dietary strategies and lifestyle tips provided, you are taking a significant step toward achieving optimal health and well-being.

Embrace the changes, remain committed, and enjoy the renewed energy and vitality that come from nurturing your adrenals.

Thank you for choosing the Adrenal Reset Diet for Beginners as your guide. Here's to your continued health and vitality!